Hypothyroidism

The Hypothyroidism Solution

Hypothyroidism Natural Treatment and Hypothyroidism Diet for Under Active Or Slow Thyroid, Causing Weight Loss Problems, Fatigue, Cardiovascular Disease, Hair Nail And Skin Problems, Depression, Menstrual Problems, Recurrent Infections And Much More

By John McArthur and Cheri Merz

Copyright

ISBN-13:978-1495308468
ISBN-10:1495308464

Natural Health Magazine

www.naturalhealthmagazine.net

The information in this book is provided for educational and information purposes only. It is not intended to be used as medical advice or as a substitute for treatment by a doctor or healthcare provider.

The information and opinions contained in this publication are believed to be accurate based on the information available to the author. However, the contents have not been evaluated by the U.S. Food and Drug Administration and are not intended to diagnose, treat, cure or prevent disease.

The author and publisher are not responsible for the use, effectiveness or safety of any procedure or treatment mentioned in this book. The publisher is not responsible for errors and omissions.

Warning

All treatment of any medical condition (without exception) must always be done under supervision of a qualified medical professional. The fact that a substance is "natural" does not necessarily mean that it has no side effects or interaction with other medications.

Medical professionals are qualified and experienced to give advice on side effects and interactions of all types of medication.

Table of Contents

Foreword

Being diagnosed with hypothyroidism means that your thyroid gland is slow or underactive and is failing to make enough hormones required to regulate metabolic processes, including growth and energy expenditure.

A few of the common symptoms are; fatigue, depression, weight gain, difficulty losing weight, cold intolerance, excessive sleepiness, dry, coarse hair, constipation, dry skin, muscle cramps, increased cholesterol levels, decreased concentration, vague aches and pains, and swelling of the legs.

As you can see, the symptoms of hypothyroidism are wide ranging and often very subtle. The symptoms can mimic the symptoms of many other conditions and in many cases doctors just attribute it to aging. Mild hypothyroidism may have no visible signs or symptoms and the symptoms only become more obvious as the condition worsens. The most common complaints are related to a metabolic slowing of the body.

The problem is that those symptoms can also be an indication of other ailments and are not exclusively related to hypothyroidism. Conventional doctors rely only on certain blood tests to determine hypothyroidism but it has been proven over and over again that those blood tests are not reliable and not sensitive enough. Because of the poor quality and insensitivity of the conventional tests, millions of people suffer from undiagnosed hypothyroidism. This is a cause for great concern because hypothyroidism is the pre-cursor of many life threatening conditions i.e. heart disease.

In this book you will find a number of easy tests, some of which you can do from home, which will help you diagnose hypothyroidism much earlier and more accurately than conventional methods.

The conventional treatment is lifelong hormone replacement therapy with drugs. The prescription drugs have serious side effects and you need to ask yourself – Do I want to explore a natural alternative before committing to a lifetime of medication?

The natural treatment options described in this book will have no side effects, will do you no harm and will improve your overall wellbeing and quality of life.

Even in the circumstances where you have to take drugs, following the natural regime described in this book will support your thyroid and do you a lot of good.

John McArthur

Introduction to the thyroid

A short biology lesson

Your thyroid is an endocrine gland, located at the base of the neck below the larynx (Adam's apple). It is shaped like a butterfly, with two wing-shaped lobes that are connected in turn by a small area called the isthmus. Endocrine glands, including the thyroid, produce substances called hormones that are essential to life and health. These hormones are carried in the blood and other circulatory systems and function to keep your entire 'engine' running correctly.

Your thyroid is controlled by your pituitary gland, which you may recall from your high school health or science class is the 'master' endocrine gland. It acts to regulate other glands in the endocrine system, using stimulating hormones to control how much hormone is produced and circulated within the blood by the other glands. The pituitary secretes thyrotropin (more commonly called Thyroid Stimulating Hormone or TSH) to regulate the hormones produced by the thyroid.

Your thyroid produces two primary hormones. The first is thyroxine, which is produced in greater quantity but is nine times less active than the other. The other is called tri-iodothyronine.

Fortunately, there is a simpler way to refer to them, based on the number of iodine atoms they have. Thyroxine is also known as T4 because of its four iodine atoms; and tri-iodothyronine is known as T3 for its three iodine atoms. A large portion of the T4 that your thyroid produces is converted to T3 by enzymes that remove one iodine atom. You might wonder, if T3 is both more active and T4 is converted to it anyway, what is the purpose of T4 at all? T4 can be considered a pre-hormone, or a raw materials supply from which T3 can also be made when required. It also turns out that T4 more readily passes through the blood/brain barrier than T3, and is then converted to the T3 that the brain requires for optimal function.

Both thyroid hormones have a profound effect on your metabolism. Do you have trouble gaining weight? Chances are you have a high metabolism that burns through the fuel you consume in the form of food rather than storing any. The opposite is true if you have a low metabolism, and both are affected by the amount of T3 and T4 that are circulating in your blood. The more hormone circulating, the higher your metabolism.

What can go wrong with the thyroid?

We have already seen that the endocrine system is quite complex. A malfunction in any of the glands can cause that gland not to do its job. Malfunctions can be the result of injury, improper nutrition, illness or can even be congenital.

There are two main conditions that result from a malfunction of the thyroid gland, the first being hypothyroidism (that is, to little thyroid hormone circulating in the blood)—the subject of this book—and hyperthyroidism (too much thyroid hormone circulating in the blood). However, there are a number of causes for each of those conditions.

For example, we already know that thyroid hormones contain iodine. Lack of iodine in our diets, or an improper balance, can interfere particularly with the thyroid's job of producing thyroid hormone. We need about 150 micrograms of iodine a day to maintain proper thyroid function. In some areas of the world, there is a lack of iodine even in the soil, and iodine deficiencies are common. That is not the case in the US, where in addition to a sufficient amount in the soil in most areas, we also have access to many foods containing iodine, including seafood and iodized salt. The result of insufficient iodine in the diet is an enlargement of the thyroid gland, commonly called goiter. When the pituitary sends TSH to the thyroid to stimulate production of more T3 and T4, but there is insufficient iodine for the gland to manufacture the hormone, the gland works harder and harder to respond, causing the swelling. Goiter can also be caused by other thyroid problems. Goiter with iodine insufficiency as the cause is uncommon in the US today.

Other conditions of the thyroid are nodules, which are thickened areas or lumps in the gland itself, and cancer. Nodules can be 'hot' areas of over-active thyroid cells, which lead to hyperthyroidism, or can be 'cold'. Cold nodules are usually of no harm, but about 20% are cancerous. Thyroid cancer is uncommon, and is readily treatable, but like any cancer requires that the sufferer receive treatment sooner rather than later.

Because the endocrine system is so complex, it is sometimes difficult to determine which condition you might have that has caused the other to occur. An analogy would be the link between illness and depression. Are you depressed because you are ill, or are you ill because you are depressed and are therefore not taking care of yourself properly? As we explore hypothyroidism and its underlying causes, remember that there may be no one answer, but a multitude of areas where small changes could mean better health for you.

How hypothyroidism impacts your daily life

Anyone who has ever been overweight knows the fatigue, sluggishness and general malaise of carrying excess pounds.

Hypothyroidism not only creates these same primary symptoms, but by causing a low metabolism also compounds the problem—making it very difficult to lose weight or not to gain it in the first place. The quality of your life with hypothyroidism can be severely diminished as you experience:

Fatigue, Sluggishness, lethargy, trouble waking up or perceived need for more sleep, Weight gain, General malaise or lack of motivation to exercise or move, Cold extremities or heightened sensitivity to cold, Depression, Brain fog, Menstrual problems, such as irregular or heavy menses, Recurrent infections and more.

The reason for so many and varied symptoms is that hypothyroidism affects every cell in your body, so that each cell's function is impacted. To understand your symptoms, it may be most useful if we catalog the effect of hypothyroidism on each body system.

Metabolic system

The thyroid has been called your gas pedal. Too much, and your metabolism runs too fast, too little, and it runs too slow.

What we mean by too slow in hypothyroidism is that the rate of utilization of your body's fuels (fat, protein and carbohydrate) is slowed. This has the consequence that your body stores unused fuels in the form of fat and the blood lipids cholesterol and

15

triglycerides. Of course you are probably aware that elevated levels of the latter are implicated in heart disease and stroke. In fact, studies have confirmed that a group of people with hypothyroidism will have a higher than average rate of atherosclerosis (caused by deposits of blood lipids inside artery walls) than a control group of individuals without hypothyroidism

As you can see, low thyroid function can be at the root of the breakdown of a chain of bodily function that is important to survival. In addition, hypothyroidism has been shown to increase capillary permeability to protein, a condition that can lead to slow lymphatic drainage and edema. Finally, another consequence of slow metabolism is the very uncomfortable state of always having cold hands and feet.

Endocrine system

The endocrine system is a tightly-linked system of glands that secrete hormones necessary for bodily function. You could think of it as a system of checks and balances, where some hormones are responsible to stimulate the production of others, and in turn monitor those others to determine whether to turn themselves on or off.

When the system gets out of balance as in hypothyroidism, a number of consequences appear that seriously affect the quality of your life. Constipation and impaired kidney function are common. Hypothyroidism has been shown to decrease libido in both men and women, to interfere with the menstrual cycle in women by causing both heavier and longer periods and a shorter time between periods. Fertility is greatly affected, as it is more difficult for the hypothyroid woman to become pregnant or to carry that pregnancy to a normal conclusion. Miscarriages and premature births are common, and stillbirths are not uncommon. Perhaps the most devastating of all consequences is potential brain damage to the baby in utero during a pregnant woman's prolonged (and typically worsening because of the strain of the pregnancy) overt hypothyroidism.

Cardiovascular

As we have already seen, hypothyroidism leads to hardening of the arteries (atherosclerosis) due to increased cholesterol and triglycerides circulating in the blood and being deposited inside the artery walls. It can also cause high blood pressure (hypertension), reduce heart rate and impair or reduce the function of the heart. Shortness of breath is a common feature of hypothyroidism.

Musculoskeletal

Hypothyroidism can lead to a general feeling of muscular weakness or stiffness, muscular or joint pain or tenderness.

Hair, skin and nails

Individuals with hypothyroidism typically have very dry hair, skin and nails. Hair may be very coarse or brittle and frequently shows signs of thinning. The outer third of the eyebrows may thin to the point of nonexistence. Skin might be so dry as to be superficially covered with what appear to be fine scales. These individuals also typically have dry, thin and brittle nails, which might exhibit transverse grooves.

Psychological

It is a particularly cruel trait of hypothyroidism that the brain appears to be quite sensitive to its effects. Depression, weakness and fatigue can be some of the first signs, followed in more overt cases by difficulty concentrating and forgetfulness (often called brain fog). The cruel part is that individuals, especially women, presenting with these symptoms and a host of others are often dismissed as hypochondriacs by doctors whose tests have failed to identify hypothyroidism. Not only do these individuals not get the treatment they need to avoid ever-worsening illness, but they are made to believe 'it's in your head,' further alienating them from friends and family who do not understand why they do not just 'get over it' or 'shake it off.'

You will notice that many of these symptoms can occur with other disorders; for example, fibromyalgia and chronic fatigue syndrome both duplicate the more debilitating symptoms in this list. Some of these symptoms can also be primary disorders in themselves; all of which makes both diagnosing and treating hypothyroidism somewhat challenging. Later we will have some suggestions for how to advocate for your own health with the knowledge you will gain from this book.

Let's start by learning more about hypothyroidism.

Hypothyroidism in more detail

In the most simple terms, hypothyroidism is the condition of having too little thyroid hormone circulating in the blood. It can also be described as having a slow or underactive thyroid. However, there are several terms that are used to describe hypothyroidism both from the perspective of how severe it is and in terms of what caused it. Throughout this book we may use some of those terms, so it behooves us to define them for you as we get started.

Terms of severity

Overt hypothyroidism refers to a condition that is easily diagnosed by the least sensitive, most common type of test. It is relatively severe, requiring treatment to avoid progression to the most critical of the grades of hypothyroidism and eventual coma or death.

Subclinical hypothyroidism refers to the condition of having some or all thyroid hormones within the accepted normal range, yet continuing to exhibit many symptoms of an underactive thyroid that are alleviated by thyroid hormone replacement therapy. We will see that this is one of the most problematic areas in diagnosis and treatment.

Myxedema or myxedema coma is loss of brain function as a result of longstanding severe hypothyroidism and is life threatening. Fortunately it is rare for hypothyroidism to be undetected for long enough to result in myxedema, but is seen in the elderly (particularly elderly women) and often in the winter months when extreme temperatures play a role.

Terms of origin

Primary hypothyroidism occurs when the thyroid is unable to produce the amount of thyroid hormone that the pituitary directs it to make. In other words, primary hypothyroid means there is something wrong with the thyroid gland itself.

There are three grades of primary hypothyroidism, measured by thyroid hormone levels. Grade one primary hypothyroidism is diagnosed when the serum FT4 level (and possibly total T3 or FT3 is below normal and TSH is very much above normal. Grade two is diagnosed when the T3 and T4 levels are within the lower half of normal but the TSH is above normal. Grade three is recognized or treated by only some doctors in the US, and is diagnosed, if at all, by a high-normal reading of a specific sub-set of TSH hormone.

Only 5% of doctors in the US treat grade three primary hypothyroidism, which in terms of severity would be considered subclinical.

Secondary hypothyroidism occurs when the pituitary gland fails to direct the thyroid to produce adequate levels of thyroid hormone.

Tertiary hypothyroidism originates one step further removed, in the failure of the hypothalamus, which governs pituitary activity. This type may also be called central hypothyroidism.

Related terms

Hyperthyroidism is essentially the opposite of hypothyroidism. Simply, it is a condition caused by an overactive thyroid, producing too much thyroid hormone. Hyperthyroidism causes the opposite effect on the metabolism, making it difficult to gain weight, or causing symptoms such as nervousness, anxiety, abnormal sensitivity to heat, rapid pulse and tremor.

Hypoparathyroidism/hyperparathyroidism. Four very small glands called parathyroid glands are located around the thyroid in the throat. The prefix 'para' means near—so these glands are near the thyroid and are part of the endocrine system. The main function of the parathyroid glands is to make the parathyroid hormone (PTH). This hormone regulates blood borne calcium, phosphorus and magnesium and also the amount of these minerals deposited in your bones. Calcium and phosphorus are crucial for healthy bones. Blood-borne calcium is also needed for muscle and nerve cell functioning. When calcium levels in the blood are too low, the parathyroid glands release extra PTH, which releases calcium from the bones and stimulates calcium reabsorption in the kidney. On the other hand, if the level of calcium in the blood is too high, the glands lower hormone production. Problems can occur if the parathyroid glands are underactive or overactive, causing similar symptoms to hyperthyroidism and hypothyroidism respectively. Causes include those related to the respective thyroid disorders and damage or surgery to the thyroid itself, as well as congenital lack of the parathyroid glands.

However, all these term definitions, while technically correct, give us no information about why the systems fail, ultimately leading to low (or high) levels of thyroid hormone. The underlying reasons are varied, and fall generally into categories relating to illness, injury or damage caused by external circumstances, congenital or dietary.

Illness and thyroid

A number of illnesses can have a debilitating effect on the thyroid. The most common of these is actually a group of illnesses, known as autoimmune disorders. The thyroid is very sensitive to these disorders where your own immune system begins attacking a normal part of your body in error; in this case, your thyroid. Autoimmune disorders of the thyroid include autoimmune thyroiditis, which is also called Hashimoto's Disease or chronic lymphocytic thyroidosis. Autoimmune thyroiditis is generally hereditary, although its progression can be impacted by environmental factors such as iodine consumption, certain drugs, infections and gender. Autoimmune thyroiditis affects women more commonly than men, and often begins with pregnancy, shortly after delivery or with menopause. As with many other disorders that are autoimmune in nature, your chances of developing autoimmune thyroiditis are higher if you already have other autoimmune disorders.

Another form of autoimmune hypothyroidism is atrophic thyroiditis. Atrophic thyroiditis occurs when the thyroid shrinks and stops making thyroid hormone in response to the immune system's attack. In both cases, the end result is a thyroid gland that is unable to meet the body's demand for thyroid hormone.

Thyroiditis is an inflammation of the thyroid gland, caused either by an autoimmune disorder as explained above, or by a viral infection. It can express itself slowly over a number of years, gradually reducing the supply of thyroid hormone in a subtle, even symptomless manner. It can also be the result of a swift attack of illness. In the case of a swift attack, thyroiditis can cause the thyroid to 'dump' its entire supply of T3 and T4 thyroid hormone at once, briefly creating a hyperthyroid condition, but reverting to hypothyroidism when the hormone supply has been completely depleted. Most patients with viral hypothyroiditis recover their thyroid function, but approximately 25% of autoimmune hypothyroiditis patients will have permanent hypothyroidism.

Less common but still worth mentioning are rare illnesses that deposit substances in the thyroid, which in turn interfere with thyroid function. Amyloidosis, for example, can deposit amyloid protein; sarcoidosis can deposit granulomas; and hemochromatosis can deposit iron.

Injury or damage to the thyroid

Because the pituitary gland regulates the thyroid, injury to the pituitary can result in the wrong instructions being given to the thyroid, producing either too little or too much thyroid hormone.

Tumors, traumatic injury, radiation or surgery can damage the pituitary in this way.

Likewise, surgical therapy for Graves disease ('hot' nodules of overactive thyroid cells) and radiation for thyroid cancer, Hodgkin's lymphoma or other cancers of the head or neck can both completely destroy the thyroid. Even partial removal of a cancerous thyroid gland can leave too little of the gland to support normal thyroid function. Of course, this type of damage is irreversible and therefore causes permanent hypothyroidism.

Medicines can also damage thyroid function. Amiodarone, interleukin-2, interferon alpha, lithium and some treatments for multiple myeloma (thalidomide) are all known to be able to interfere with the thyroid gland. Patients with a genetic tendency to autoimmune thyroiditis are more likely to have it triggered by these medicines.

Fortunately less common, heavy metal toxicity or overexposure to environmental toxins is very damaging to the entire endocrine system, including the thyroid.

Congenital

Sadly, some babies are born with thyroid problems ranging from ectopic thyroid (having the thyroid gland in the wrong place) to partially-formed thyroid to no thyroid at all. Some babies have thyroid cells or enzymes that do not function properly. In some cases, the thyroid retains enough function to supply sufficient thyroid hormone for a while and then the individual becomes hypothyroid; while in others there is too little thyroid function to sustain normal development. In the latter case, immediate thyroid hormone replacement therapy is essential to prevent brain damage or even death. Because this is such a serious condition, all babies born under medical care in the US are now tested for it.

Diet and thyroid

The most important dietary concern in hypothyroidism is the consumption of iodine. The thyroid gland requires iodine to make thyroid hormone. Iodine is consumed in foods, mainly chicken, pork, beef, dairy products, fish, and iodized salt. The iodine is then incorporated by the thyroid gland into the thyroid hormones T3 and T4, which as you will recall are named to match the number of iodine atoms in each hormone. The correct amount of iodine is vital to keeping hormone production in balance.

Worldwide, particularly in underdeveloped countries where people may not get enough iodine in their diet, iodine deficiency is the most prevalent cause of hypothyroidism; however, it is a rare cause in the U.S. Consuming too much iodine can also cause or worsen hypothyroidism in a rebound effect. The major source of too much iodine is dietary supplements containing a type of seaweed called kelp, often touted as helping people lose weight. Other sources of too much iodine are x-ray dyes, some medicines and some older cough medicines known as expectorants.

Other dietary concerns are foods that, while excess consumption of them does not cause hypothyroidism, can interfere with optimal thyroid function. We will explore this topic in a later section.

Who is at risk of hypothyroidism?

A better question would be who isn't at risk! The short answer to that question is African-Americans, but only to the extent that the risk is lower.

Hypothyroidism is one of the most common thyroid disorders, affecting a broad spectrum of the world's population. It is no respecter of age, race or socioeconomic class. The American Association of Clinical Endocrinologists (AACE) estimates that as many as 10% of Americans have thyroid disease. That is more than the number with cancer and diabetes combined. In other words, millions have underactive thyroid, many of those receive inadequate treatment, and as many as half of them do not even know they have the condition. That is because they go undiagnosed by the conventional testing methods.

Another way to look at it is what are the risk factors?

The most common cause of hypothyroidism is autoimmune disorder, as discussed above. Accordingly, risk factors for autoimmune hypothyroidism begin with family history. If you have a close relative with autoimmune hypothyroidism, your risk of developing it is greater.

Next is age. Although hypothyroidism can start at any age, the risk grows as you grow older. Females more commonly develop it than males, especially in the younger years. Risk for males begins to overtake that of females as they age. Women are particularly vulnerable at times of hormonal upheaval, such as during pregnancy, after delivery, or at menopause.

Some estimates put the incidence of subclinical or undiagnosed hypothyroidism among women over age 60 as high as 20% of the population in the US.

Finally, race plays a part, as Caucasians and Asians have a higher risk than African-Americans.

Aside from issues of age, race and family history, other risks include having any other type of autoimmune disorder, which can interfere with the endocrine system and therefore weaken the thyroid. Although there is a long list of autoimmune disorders, these few are examples but not an exhaustive list of those that can trigger autoimmune hypothyroidism: rheumatoid arthritis, multiple sclerosis, Addison's disease, pernicious anemia.

Who else is at risk? People with chromosomal abnormalities, such as Down syndrome or Turner syndrome are vulnerable to hypothyroidism along with a spectrum of other disorders associated with their condition. Bi-polar disorder also leaves one vulnerable to hypothyroidism, whether as a primary trigger or because of the medications typically used to treat the condition, such as lithium.

Signs and symptoms of hypothyroidism

We have already listed a number of symptoms that impact the daily quality of life with hypothyroidism. Here, however, is a more exhaustive list of signs and symptoms:

- Fatigue
- Depression
- Weight gain or inability/difficulty to lose weight
- Dry skin, yellow skin
- Intolerance of cold
- Hair loss or coarse hair
- Hoarse voice
- Constipation
- Fluid retention
- Decreased concentration, forgetfulness and other evidence of intellectual impairment
- Facial puffiness
- Macroglossia (unusual enlargement of the tongue)
- Slow speech
- Reflex delay in the relaxation phase
- Ataxia (lack of voluntary control of muscle movement)

- Irregular or heavy menses and infertility
- Myalgias
- Hyperlipidemia (high cholesterol)
- Bradycardia (slow heartbeat) and hypothermia (abnormally low basal temperature)
- Myxedema (critical clinical hypothyroidism requiring immediate medical intervention to prevent brain damage or death in adults)
- Anemia

Naturally, some of these symptoms are of more concern than others, but none are without discomfort and none have a salutary impact on daily life.

What is the effect of hypothyroidism?

Clearly, the degree of incapacitation from hypothyroidism is related to the severity of the condition and whether it is controlled by treatment, which is readily available. At the subclinical end of the spectrum, you might notice a few uncomfortable symptoms and perhaps think that they are associated with some other condition. Perhaps you have slowly gained weight, and now believe that your fatigue and sluggishness are simply due to the extra pounds. An older woman might attribute the gradual loss of the outer third of her eyebrows to age, observing other older women with thinning eyebrows. A younger woman might believe her heavy menstrual periods are genetic, hearing her mother tell of her own heavy periods. The lack of specific symptoms, that is, symptoms always occurring with hypothyroidism and never occurring with any other condition alone, creates great difficulty in diagnosing hypothyroidism at this end of the spectrum.

Conversely, critical hypothyroidism, most likely stemming from a more rapid onset such as might happen with a viral infection or pregnancy can also have symptoms that are more readily attributable to the correct cause. As an example, Victoria [pseudonym] experienced rapid swelling of the thyroid gland during pregnancy, when her previously controlled hypothyroidism required more and more support because of the demands of the pregnancy on her body. Not only was the swelling visible, but the enlarging thyroid gland impinged on her larynx, causing hoarseness and pain. It was never questioned that there could be another cause besides uncontrolled hypothyroidism, and indeed increasing the dose of her medication took care of the problem, which reverted to its pre-pregnancy level after delivery.

Whether the impact is relatively mild or severe, hypothyroidism is a serious condition, requiring attention. Extended periods of subclinical hypothyroidism may be to blame for or may exacerbate the obesity epidemic in the US, with its consequences of heart disease, stroke and even some forms of cancer. These so-called lifestyle diseases taken as a group are the reason for the healthcare crisis the American economy is facing today. We might ask, "Why is there such a high incidence of undiagnosed hypothyroidism?" The answer to that question lies in how hypothyroidism is diagnosed.

How is hypothyroidism diagnosed?

Conventional methods of diagnosis:

As we have noted before, there are no symptoms of hypothyroidism that are characteristic of the condition alone. Undiagnosed hypothyroidism may be the underlying cause of any number of health problems that have been non-responsive to treatment. In fact, the patient may attribute her symptoms to another cause and fail to seek medical assistance at all, or seek assistance for an unrelated condition that presents with the same or similar symptoms.

Compounding the problem, the long list of symptoms that may occur with hypothyroidism are seldom all present in the same individual. Those that are typically present, like dry skin, may send the patient to a dermatologist, who may treat the symptom without seeking the cause. Or heavy menstrual periods may cause the patient to see a gynecologist, who might treat that symptom with birth control pills to 'regulate' it, again without seeking the underlying cause. Like the seven blind men trying to describe an elephant, it would be difficult for a doctor to pinpoint hypothyroidism as a diagnosis if presented with only one or two related symptoms.

What is insidious about this state of affairs is that, in addition to the consequences already discussed, long-term subclinical hypothyroidism can 'wear out' or fatigue the endocrine system, leading to irreversible hypothyroidism. Similarly to the mechanism that causes the progression from insulin resistance to Type II diabetes, subclinical hypothyroidism can lead to the more serious illness that cannot be ignored.

Once hypothyroidism is suspected, there is typically just one test that most doctors will perform, which evaluates TSH levels. More often than not, if the TSH level is normal, that will be the end of any investigation of hypothyroidism as the cause of the symptoms. However, having normal TSH levels does not necessarily mean that the thyroid is functioning normally. This is undoubtedly the cause of the high incidence of underactive thyroid going undiagnosed. Several quotes from medical journals and highly-respected endocrinologists are included in Appendix A to support this statement.

To advocate for your own health, you should know that there are several other tests available to help in the diagnosis of thyroid problems. These include free T3, free T4, and reverse T3, for a complete thyroid function panel. Thyroid antibody tests support the diagnosis of hypothyroidism; however, elevated levels of thyroid antibodies predict with high correlation the incidence of developing thyroid disease even when more conventional tests produce results within the normal range. Thyroid antibody tests are for thyroid peroxidase antibodies (TPO Ab) which are sometimes referred to as Microsomal antibodies, and thyroglobulin antibodies (Tg Ab). Women may also receive valuable information with a hormone profile: E2, Progesterone, Testosterone, DHEAS, Cortisol (and E1 & E3 if possible).

You should also be aware that the American Association of Clinical Endocrinologists (AACE) has recently lowered their recommendations for acceptable TSH values to help diagnose more people with low thyroid function. TSH is inversely related to T3 and T4; that is, the more TSH, the lower the T3 and T4 levels; therefore, lowering the acceptable TSH values would detect what have previously been subclinical hypothyroidism; nevertheless, patients who see, for example, general practitioners or internists rather than endocrinologists for their symptoms may still go undiagnosed because the more sensitive tests are not frequently ordered.

John V. Dommisse, MD, MBChB, FRCP(C), in an article for www.ThyroidScience.com, has stated that, astoundingly, "...a free T3 level by the tracer-dialysis method, the only accurate indicator of this exclusively-active hormone's function, is rarely obtained."

(Emphasis ours.) You might come to the conclusion that the majority of the medical profession is near-criminally negligent in regard to diagnosing and treating subclinical hypothyroidism and you might not be wrong.

In addition to the tests mentioned above, there are a number of related illnesses and disorders that can either be the proximate cause of hyperthyroidism, or can be caused or exacerbated by having hyperthyroidism. While it is beyond the scope of this book to explore these illnesses and their treatments (both conventional and alternative) in detail, be particularly aware of the need to assess your health regarding diabetes, inflammation or unhealthy liver. Always use a qualified health care professional to assist you in being tested for these conditions, and note that there are many natural therapies that can treat, alleviate or support function in these areas as well as in hypothyroidism alone.

What's wrong with conventional diagnosis only?

Patients and clinicians alike have observed that conventional diagnosis only is inadequate, for a number of reasons beginning with the fact that often only the TSH test is used. As we have seen, the TSH test does not tell the whole story. Countless patients with normal TSH values have been told their thyroid is not the problem, yet still have numerous symptoms pointing to hypothyroidism. Certainly the symptoms do not point only to hypothyroidism, and that is where a doctor with both the experience and the patience to further explore is invaluable.

A second reason that so-called 'normal' TSH levels do not tell the whole story is that the range of 'normal' is quite broad. Not only that, but an individual's TSH levels vary throughout the course of even a day, as well as being affected by factors such as environmental conditions, prescription drugs, other illness and even other hormones being produced by the body at any given time. A test provides a snapshot of the individual's TSH values at a given moment in time, and has nothing at all to say about whether the level measured is normal for that individual, even if it falls within the spectrum of 'normal' that is currently defined. Perhaps it is at the low end of the range considered normal, but the individual previously, before developing the symptoms that drove her to seek medical attention, had levels at the high end of the range. One of the acute causes of hypothyroidism, say viral infection, may have caused those levels to drop, but not to defined clinical levels. That individual is poorly served by being told that her thyroid is not the problem, and may in fact continue to decline when a timely medical intervention of thyroid replacement hormone or nutritional support would have restored her thyroid to health.

The definition of normal TSH values as well as that for other thyroid hormones has actually changed as medical knowledge advances, too. And let us not forget human error. It has been stated that results of the same sample, divided and sent to more than one laboratory, can vary by as much as 50%.

The bottom line is that, as patients, we must become our own advocates. Rather than accepting a label of hypochondriac (not unusual, especially for women presenting with a spectrum of vague, non-measurable and non-specific complaints) we must press for a more accurate and individualized diagnosis. Often, diagnosis becomes a process of eliminating the other causes for each symptom; however a knowledgeable doctor might cut to the chase by offering a low therapeutic dose of thyroid replacement therapy to see if the symptoms begin to improve.

If you have not yet found a doctor who will work with you to get to the root cause of your symptoms, you might find the next section quite valuable.

Alternative methods of diagnosing hypothyroidism

Prior to the current conventional medical tests, there were a number of ways to determine whether hypothyroidism was a likely culprit for your symptoms. Although your doctor may not value them, you can use these same methods today to make a determination whether to push for the more expensive and less common laboratory tests, or to decide whether to use natural methods to support your thyroid function.

The first idea is to think back and try to remember whether this is a new symptom, or whether you have always had it. Generally, the longer you have had the symptom, the less likely that you have hypothyroidism. Untreated clinical hypothyroidism becomes worse and worse and the metabolism becomes slower and slower, eventually leading to death within ten to fifteen years. One would hope that long before this occurs; even conventional tests would have uncovered the condition. However, there is an argument to be made for the idea that long-term symptoms could be related to a slightly underactive thyroid that could still be improved by supporting it with nutrients that improve thyroid function.

The basal body temperature test

A strong symptom of hypothyroidism can be measured quantitatively, which can help diagnose it. It is common for a person with hypothyroidism to have a low basal temperature (that is, the temperature of your body at rest), as much as 2 to 4 degrees below normal. Certainly that would also explain the symptom of hypersensitivity to cold - that individual is literally colder than normal, even when the air temperature is warm!

With every degree body temperature is decreased, metabolic rate is decreased by approximately 6%, which also explains the feelings of fatigue and sluggishness, as well as the weight gain associated with hypothyroidism. To detect potential hypothyroidism by use of basal body temperature, you must follow a protocol that will allow you to accurately measure your temperature upon first awakening and before getting out of bed.

You will need a glass mercury thermometer or a digital thermometer with no less than 0.5 F readings. Special basal temperature thermometers are frequently used to predict ovulation and are not only very sensitive to minor variations in temperature but are also very easy to read, so you might want to acquire one of these, available at most drugstores. Shake down the thermometer to below 95F and place it where you can reach it without moving upon awakening. Do not leave this shaking down until morning, as the movement associated with it will cause your basal body temperature to rise.

In the morning, preferably at the same time each day, place the thermometer in your armpit before moving or arising and hold it there for ten to fifteen minutes. Record the temperature and time. You should do this for three to six mornings in a row, and average the temperature. An average temperature that is significantly lower than the 97.6F to 98.2F normal temperature range could indicate hypothyroidism. A temperature that is consistently below 96F is a very good indication that you definitely have an underactive thyroid.

It should be noted that menstruating women must perform the test on the second, third, and fourth days of menstruation. Postmenopausal women or men can perform the test at any time. Note also that an electric blanket or water bed can artificially interfere with the basal temperature, so these should be avoided when performing this test. Finally, an unusually high basal temperature unrelated to an artificial heat source or fever could indicate hyperthyroidism, which also requires intervention.

The iodine tincture patch test

Another useful home test, although more subjective than the temperature test, is a quick analysis of your body's iodine levels. After applying small amounts of iodine liquid (Betadine, for example) on the skin, your body will absorb the iodine it requires; therefore if you are deficient in iodine, your skin will rapidly absorb the iodine applied on it. This typically will take place over the next eight hours; however, if your iodine levels are adequate, the iodine will not be absorbed and will leave a stain on your skin that will fade over the next few days.

At night before bedtime, apply a 2" x 2" square of iodine liquid such as Betadine to your abdomen or upper thigh. Iodine liquid is sold as an antiseptic for minor cuts and scrapes at most pharmacies. DO NOT SHOWER DIRECTLY AFTER APPLYING.

In the morning when you arise, note the color and check the answer that is most correct:

- Same color as applied (Adequate iodine levels)
- Pale Yellow (Borderline iodine levels)
- Grayish colored (Iodine deficiency)
- No color left (Iodine deficiency)

If there is NO color remaining, then you may consider your test is complete. If there is ANY color remaining, continue to check the color of the patch every few hours. Make a note of the time when the color is entirely gone. If the color still remains at bedtime, the test is complete. The color will fade over the next few days

- No color by 12pm noon (Iodine deficiency)
- Color gone by 4pm (Borderline iodine levels)
- Color gone by 8pm (Adequate iodine levels)
- Color gone by bedtime (Adequate iodine levels)
- Some color remaining (Adequate iodine levels)

Remember that inadequate iodine levels are not the only cause of hypothyroidism, and in fact is a rare cause in the US. This test, therefore, does not rule out hypothyroidism, only inadequate iodine levels. It is useful because if you are one of the rare individuals with inadequate iodine levels, you are most definitely at risk for developing hypothyroidism if not already suffering from it and should seek medical attention right away, in addition to utilizing the natural methods that are presented in later chapters.

You should be aware, however, that once the thyroid stops working properly, supplementing specifically with more iodine will not help and can actually be harmful. In fact, iodine overdose can actually lead to hypothyroidism. Signs of overdose include nausea, diarrhea, skin rash, fever, joint pains, trouble breathing, facial swelling or swelling of the throat, metallic taste, burning mouth, sore teeth and gums, head cold symptoms and enlarged thyroid. If you suspect inadequate iodine in your system, caution would indicate that you seek medical confirmation and supplement only as directed by a doctor. If you have been supplementing iodine either as a weight-loss strategy or as a consequence of other supplementation and have any of the above symptoms, seek medical attention right away.

The reflexes test

Achilles tendon reflex can be an indicator of hypothyroidism, although the efficacy of this test is limited due to the number and variety of other conditions that can slow reflex time. With overt hypothyroidism, the relaxation phase of the reflex can be slowed.

Reflex timing is probably not something that a layman can adequately evaluate.

Swelling in the base of the neck

An underactive thyroid frequently looks swollen, but can also look normal or even undersized. Certainly if you notice that your neck is swelling at its base, or if you feel internal pressure there, a visit to your doctor would be wise.

None of these alternative methods of diagnosing hypothyroidism are now considered definitive by the medical community. All results can have other causes, or none may be present in any given case of hypothyroidism. However, if you are concerned about symptoms of hypothyroidism and have had your concerns dismissed by your physician because of a TSH test with normal values, the evidence you present for these indicators could mean the difference between being sent home as a hypochondriac and your doctor being willing to explore further with more reliable or more sensitive tests. In short, a person who is actively engaged in her own health decisions would do well to include both conventional and alternative diagnostic methods in the search for answers.

Conventional treatment methods

What conventional therapies are available to treat hypothyroidism?

Hypothyroidism is considered by the conventional medical establishment to be incurable. However, available medications that are taken every day can completely control the symptoms by replacing the hormone that the thyroid is no longer making with a synthetic form of it.

The American Association of Clinical Endocrinologists recommends treatment for patients with overt hypothyroidism characterized by a TSH level ≥10 mU/mL, and close follow-up for patients with subclinical levels. Conventional medical treatment most often means prescription of synthetic thyroxine (T4) under one of several trade names, including Synthroid, Levoxyl, Levothroid. These are levothyroxine sodium products, also called L-thyroxine, and which are also available under other names and as a generic medication.

Similarly to the T4 that your own thyroid gland makes, a dose of synthetic thyroxine continues to work in your blood for approximately a week, meaning your T4 levels stay steady, providing a constant supply of T4 to your body. You may recall that the other thyroid hormone your body requires, T3, is able to be supplied by conversion from T4. While this is the accepted treatment protocol among the mainstream medical establishment, there are a couple of other treatments that some doctors argue are more effective.

You may also recall from our previous discussion that T3 is nine times more active in the body than T4, which leads some physicians to advocate treating with both hormones. The synthetic form of T3 is called liothyronine (brand name, Cytomel). It can supplement treatment with levothyroxine or be prescribed in a time released compounded version. Treating with both synthetic hormones has been supported in research featured in the New England Journal of Medicine, but other researchers have also claimed it to be ineffective, so some controversy remains. Some practitioners believe that patients do not need T3, because the body will convert T4 into the T3 it needs. The alternative medical community believes that direct T3 supplementation is warranted by the potential of impaired conversion of T4 to T3, creating a deficiency of the latter.

In addition to synthetic thyroid hormones, another available thyroid supplement is natural, desiccated thyroid obtained from pigs (which are genetically quite similar to humans) or cows. Some clinicians believe these preparations that go by the brand names of Armour Thyroid or Thyrolar are more effective than synthetic hormone because it contains the full spectrum of thyroid hormone, beyond T3 and T4. Others believe the variable T3:T4 ratio that characterizes natural hormone could be counterproductive, even dangerous. It should be noted that among physicians who do not supplement with T3, a major reason is that overdose of T3 can cause heart palpitations and other cardiac side effects. It can also cause high T3 levels but low T4, the opposite of a normal physiological ratio, and can be dangerous to fetal development among pregnant women.

It is important to understand that thyroid hormone replacement therapy must be highly individualized and carefully monitored. Small changes in the dose or the patient can backfire, sending the patient from euthyroidism (optimal thyroid function) to hypo- or hyperthyroidism in a short period of time. For this reason, some clinicians are inclined to prescribe individually-titered doses rather than standard increments. No matter how synthetic or natural thyroid hormone is prescribed, it is essential that the patient be closely monitored and the dose adjusted accordingly. Most physicians will start with a minimal dose and increase as necessary, bearing in mind that over-medication will result in subclinical or overt hyperthyroidism.

Pros and cons of thyroid hormone replacement

Among the benefits of conventional medical treatment are that replacement therapy is relatively simple to evaluate and adjust. Compliance is fairly easy - just take your medication as prescribed. But with this ease comes very real risk of unintended consequences ranging from over treatment to the side effects associated with the drugs themselves.

Side effects of levothyroxine sodium

Common side effects of T4 replacement therapy are experienced typically with therapeutic overmedication, and reflect the symptoms of hyperthyroidism. They include increased appetite, weight loss, insomnia, anxiety, heat intolerance, increase in bowel frequency or diarrhea, heart palpitations, high blood pressure, tachycardia, angina, and menstrual irregularities. Among these, the cardiovascular-related side effects can exacerbate cardiac disease. Other side effects are either rare or transient, including changes in symptoms of diabetes, adrenal cortex insufficiency, seizures, hair loss or other dermatologic symptoms and potentially risk of osteoporosis, although the latter has seen conflicting study results.

Side effects of liothyronine

All of the side effects reported with therapeutic overdose of synthetic T4 hormone are also reported for therapeutic overdose of synthetic T3. Add to the above, excessive sweating, as well as nervousness, irritability and tremor. There have been serious allergic reactions to liothyronine as well. Patients are directed to get emergency medical help if they experience symptoms including difficult breathing; swelling of the face, lips, tongue, or throat or hives.

Side effects of desiccated thyroid

There seems to be some controversy in the literature regarding the variability of hormone ratio in this natural hormone replacement (natural as opposed to the synthetic preparations that is). Many successful practitioners prefer it for its complete spectrum of thyroid hormone, which includes trace substances beyond T3 and T4.

Others disregard it because it is 'antiquated', variable in strength or for other reasons, one of which might be the objection of vegans and vegetarians to ingesting animal product. However, the side effects, as with the previously mentioned drugs, are mainly the same symptoms of hyperthyroidism stemming from therapeutic overdose and, more rarely, allergy. Practitioners who take the view that it is more natural seem to believe it is also easier to avoid therapeutic overdose with this preparation.

Alternative or natural methods of hypothyroidism treatment

Natural methods of treatment for any illness or condition rely on a multi-faceted approach of lifestyle changes, nutrition, environmental changes and various naturopathic disciplines. Because hypothyroidism in its worst incarnation is life-threatening, we must caution you to apply the following information very carefully, and preferably after seeking opinions from both conventional and alternative caregivers.

It is neither possible nor advisable to self-diagnose or self-treat overt hypothyroidism. Nor is a natural remedy necessarily safe or free from side effects just because it is natural. That said, many of the recommendations to follow are widely accepted as healthful whether or not an individual can improve subclinical hypothyroidism by adopting them. The author of this book is not a physician of any sort, and can only express opinion based on research and personal experience. This book, therefore, is not offered as medical advice, and any use you make of it must be at your own risk and with full awareness that failure to consult medical professionals could have very adverse consequences.

What natural treatments are available for hypothyroidism?

There are a number of foods, herbs, and micro-nutrients such as vitamins and minerals that either support or interfere with thyroid function. If you are suffering from symptoms of hypothyroidism, chances are your diet has not been optimal for best health or you may have been consuming very healthful foods in quantities that can unfortunately interfere with thyroid function. We will explore those in detail shortly. Other food considerations are foods that have been enhanced with artificial hormones, chiefly meat, chicken, dairy products and eggs, although genetically-modified foods may also be suspect. Any time you consume a food with artificial hormones, you risk interfering with the proper function of hormone synthesis in your own body. Choose organic and free-range foods when possible check labels for added synthetic hormones and avoid them when possible. Unfortunately, there is no requirement for GMO identification, but there is plenty of information available about the food companies who use them on the internet these days for those who want to avoid them.

Start with a good detox

Natural health caregivers and people who have begun to pay close attention to the way their bodies work in their thousands have begun over the past few years to sing the praises of cleansing, or detoxifying, their digestive systems, livers and indeed all their tissues, from the bad habits of years. There is some evidence that if you want to change your health via your nutrition, it makes sense to do some housekeeping in the form of a cleanse or detoxification so that your new diet has less to do in the way of corrective measures and can immediately begin supporting good health.

You may use any cleanse or detox protocol you have previously found effective, or you may use the protocol in the following paragraphs. Before you do either, consult with your doctor to make sure that no part of it will worsen your illness. Some of the foods we will recommend contradict our later advice regarding foods to eat or avoid with hypothyroidism. Chances are you have been consuming these foods, and we suggest you begin to follow that later advice after a nine-day detox diet that will ready your body for better health. If, however, you have already received a diagnosis of Hashimoto's disease (autoimmune hypothyroidism), any other autoimmune disease, acute hypothyroidism or elevated thyroid antibodies, do not follow this detox protocol but go straight to the dietary recommendations in the section for nutritional therapy.

The idea behind a detox is to supply your body with its nutritional needs while encouraging waste elimination and avoiding substances that promote a build-up of solid waste. For this reason, you will avoid all grains, particularly wheat or any product containing gluten. You will also avoid artificial preservatives and highly-processed foods such as sugar and white flour; artificial flavorings and colorings; caffeinated beverages such as coffee and black teas; dairy, nuts, and alcohol and above all, junk foods. "What CAN I eat, then?!" you might say. Read on.

Below you will find a list of suggestions for each meal of the day. Those suggestions include a couple of supportive recipes that you can make up in a big batch and have on hand for the occasions when the protocol calls for them.

Potassium soup

Start with ½ cup each of the following high-potassium vegetables, chopped:

Potato, spinach, beetroot, carrot, celery, onion, tomato, ginger

Add if desired: miso, to taste

Add to 1 quart boiling water, bring back to a simmer and simmer for ½ hour

Strain and discard vegetables

Serving = 1 cup

Detox gumbo

6 fresh tomatoes

2 onions

Parsley

Sea Salt and/or pepper to taste

In large pot, sauté above ingredients in ½ C olive oil until quite tender and beginning to brown

Add 3 C water and 5 potatoes cut in half, bring to boil and cook until potatoes begin to soften

Add 2 lbs. whole baby okra (can be canned okra)

Cook while stirring for about 15 minutes, until mixture has thickened.

Best enjoyed hot. (Some people do not appreciate the texture of boiled okra, or the texture of the thickened sauce; however this is the important part of the formula as the fiber stimulates bowel cleanse.)

Now you are prepared to enjoy the following meal plan for the next nine days, or you can extend it to 14 days if you are feeling excellent at the end of the original protocol.

You should feel more energetic, chances are you will have lost weight and/or inches, and your skin and hair should begin to look more healthy and shiny.

Hypothyroid meal plan suggestions

Breakfast

2 soft-boiled eggs or at least 3 pieces of fruit

Breakfast should be eaten within an hour of arising, or before noon.

Lunch

Choose one or two of the following, in any combination:

1 C potassium soup

1 C detox gumbo

5-7 raw vegetables in a salad

Canned fish such as tuna or salmon or organic chicken with no skin

Mid afternoon snack

1 C potassium soup

5-7 steamed vegetables

2 pieces of fruit, fruit juice or vegetable juice

As a particular treat and to add nutrients, squeeze or extract your own juices and add a shot of wheat grass, available from health stores in powder form.

Dinner

2-3 C steamed vegetables consisting of 5-7 vegetables or

1 C Detox gumbo or

Raw salad of 5-7 vegetables

plus

1 serving of a protein source the size of your palm. Choose from:

2 eggs, boiled or poached, organic or free-range

Or fish (deep-sea, such as sardines, salmon, tuna, mackerel, cod and snapper or other)

Or organic chicken or turkey (no skin)

Or legumes (chickpea, lentils, soy and soy products such as tofu)

Or vegetable patties with tofu or chickpeas

Or fish or chicken soup

Tips

Eat plenty of the suggested foods, but do not overeat. If you feel hungry between meals, two teaspoons of psyllium husks taken in a glass of water can help. Increasing your overall water intake will not only help with feeling fuller, but will also provide for even better detoxification.

Choose organic foods when possible, but if you cannot get organic, wash foods thoroughly.

If you have never completed a cleanse before, or if you are particularly toxic to begin with, you may experience uncomfortable digestive feelings, headache, fatigue or mental fogginess. These signs and symptoms are normal. It may help to start the cleanse on a weekend or when you otherwise have a couple or three days when you do not have to go to work or have other obligations.

Get plenty of rest, relaxation and sleep, particularly during the first few days. Most of these symptoms will ease or disappear within two to three days and you will begin to feel much better than you did before you started, but if they become too intense for you to function normally, please stop the cleanse at once.

You can assist your body to detoxify by taking a hot Epsom salts bath every second night, or alternatively, a sea salts bath. Feel free to add essential oils of your choice for relaxation, but do not stay in the bath excessively long as this may result in diarrhea.

You may also enhance your detox by supporting your liver function with preparations available from your health food store that include one or more of Bupleurum, Dandelion, Globe Artichoke, Schisandra or St. Mary's Thistle.

Finally, sufferers from autoimmune disorders often find that micro-organisms or parasites are a contributing factor, secreting toxins that attack your organs and glands. Addition of herbal supplements known to fight these can significantly improve your health, but you should seek the counsel of healthcare practitioners, specifically naturopaths and nutritionists, for dosage and use instructions. Herbs known to fight micro-organisms and parasites include: Barberry (Berberis vulgaris), Black Walnut (Juglans nigra), Chinese Wormwood (Artemisia annua), Citrus seed extract (Citrus paradise), Cloves (Syzgium aromaticum or Eugenia carophyllus), Echinacea (Echinacea angustifolia/purpurea), Oregano (Origanum vulgare), Thyme (Thymus vulgaris) and Wormwood (Artemisia annua).

Following the cleanse, you will want to begin to avoid foods that exacerbate thyroid malfunction and add foods that support healthy thyroid function. In the next sections we will explore those to avoid and why, as well as those to eat more of and why.

Foods to avoid and why

Even a very superficial reading of the literature will quickly find that there is a class of foods that we all think of as very healthy, and have been encouraged from our earliest years to eat, that can be nevertheless harmful or at least not supportive of thyroid health. We are referring to the cruciferous, or cabbage family of vegetables that includes cabbage, Brussels sprouts, cauliflower, kale, mustard greens and spinach. While normally very good for you, these foods contain high levels of thiourea, which is thought to interfere with thyroid function by binding the free iodine that the thyroid requires to manufacture thyroid hormone. Fruits containing the same substance include peaches, pears, apples and strawberries. Other foods that also contain high levels of thiourea are soy and peanuts, rutabaga, turnips, walnuts, and almonds.

All of the foods mentioned in the preceding paragraph are considered goitrogenic; that is, complicit in the formation of goiter, a swelling of the thyroid gland most often caused by improper thyroid function. It is a mistake to simplify the mechanism and assume that these foods actually cause hypothyroidism. In fact, once hypothyroidism is controlled, you may enjoy these foods in moderation, particularly if they are cooked, as cooking alters the compound that binds to iodine and renders it relatively harmless.

In addition to the foods containing thiourea, it is a good idea to eliminate or limit caffeine, which by stimulating the adrenal gland also alter the activity of glands further down the line in the endocrine system, thyroid included.

Foods to eat, and why

Within limits, to avoid iodine overdose, consume foods that are naturally high in iodine to provide one of the important building blocks of thyroid hormone. Foods high in iodine are fish or seafood as well as seaweed such as kelp, ararne and nori. Vegetables that are high in iodine include Swiss chard, artichokes and butter beans as well as root vegetables (such as potatoes). Seeds and nuts high in iodine include pumpkin seeds and sesame seeds (tahini). Additionally, egg yolk, lecithin, minced beef, onions, garlic, mushrooms are all high in iodine.

Tyrosine is another building block for thyroid hormone, and can be found in all protein-rich foods, especially some of the foods mentioned above as well as bananas and avocados. If you have adequate protein in your diet you should be getting enough tyrosine. Vegetarians and vegans should be especially careful to consider the quality of their protein, but it is not necessary to consume animal products to get enough protein.

Proper thyroid function requires essential fatty acids also. To provide plenty of omega 3 fatty acids in your diet, include oily fish, seeds and cold pressed oils such as flaxseed. Omega 6 fatty acids are generally not lacking in the American diet. Avoiding highly saturated fats and trans-fats is advised for all dietary concerns, however not all saturated fats are created equal. For use in cooking where a sweeter, lighter taste than olive oil is desired, consider virgin coconut oil; just steer clear of the partially-hydrogenated product. Coconut oil is thought to stimulate the thyroid, a bonus for this purpose.

The trace mineral manganese also contributes importantly to thyroid function. You can healthfully add manganese to your diet by eating nuts (pecans, Brazil nuts) and grains (barley, rye, buckwheat).

Other foods that support thyroid function include radishes, watercress, wheat germ, brewer's yeast, tropical fruits, and watermelon. Some of the literature recommends making your own watermelon juice and adding aloe vera juice for a great thyroid blend; however, consume aloe vera juice with caution as unwanted side effects are possible.

Vitamin and mineral supplements that you can use safely include 1000 mg of vitamin C per day and 100 mg of CoQ10 daily to raise energy levels. You may also want to supplement with 1-3 grams of

Siberian ginseng, a known stress-reliever. Avoid Korean ginseng if you have high blood pressure.

Thyro Complex is a formulation by naturopath Martin Budd, an established authority on thyroid health. He has spent 15 years researching the nutritional support required for healthy thyroid function, and his formula contains all the nutrients needed to help support the thyroid. Take 1-3 tablets daily 30 minutes before food. Check the ingredients and adjust other supplements to avoid taking too much of some vitamins.

A word about food sensitivities, allergies, and food-related illnesses

Proper nutritional support can be a complex subject, particularly when dealing with a condition that can be caused or exacerbated by other underlying disease process or allergies. Some of these conditions can in turn be caused or exacerbated by substances in food. A well-known example of this is celiac disease, in which gluten, a protein found in many grains, is unable to be digested and causes severe gastric distress when consumed. Gluten has also been implicated in several other complaints and even people who cannot specifically point to a particular reason for it have been known to just feel better after eliminating gluten from their diets. It may well be that eliminating gluten or other foods to which you have an allergy or sensitivity could have a positive effect on your thyroid function as well.

Your new shopping list

Eliminating foods or whole classes of food from your diet may be confusing, unpleasant and leave you feeling there is nothing you can safely eat! What follows is a grocery shopping list of thyroid-supporting foods as well as a list of food substitutes for foods that are common allergy culprits.

Foods to buy and eat more of:

- Fish/Seafood
- Minced beef
- Eggs
- High Protein Grains
- Swiss chard
- Butterbeans
- Carrots
- Dark green and yellow vegetables except those that are goitrogenic
- Radishes
- Potatoes
- Mushrooms
- Watercress

- Onions

- Garlic

- Tropical fruit

- Bananas

- Avocado

- Watermelon

- Pecans

- Brazil nuts

- Pumpkin seeds

- Sesame seeds

Food substitutes:

If you are sensitive to:	Substitute for:
Wheat or gluten	Quinoa, Rice, Corn, Buckwheat, Barley, Amaranth, Millet, Sorghum
Milk	Rice milk, almond milk, goat or sheep's milk
Ice Cream	Sorbet, frozen blended banana, homemade using milk substitutes
Cheese	Goat or sheep's milk cheeses
Butter	Nut butters (e.g. Nutella, almond butter), olive oil, flax oil, macadamia oil, mashed avocado, tahini, hummus, sesame oil

Sugar or sweeteners	Xylitol, agave syrup, honey, maple syrup, stevia
Chocolate	Carob

Other beneficial nutrients

Micro-nutrients, i.e., vitamins, minerals and phytochemicals play an enormous part in nutrition that is far beyond the scope of this eBook to explore fully. Nevertheless, there are some substances that have been shown to support thyroid function sufficiently to warrant a discussion of supplementation.

Iodine

Historically, iodine deficiency was one of the most common causes of hypothyroidism, and remains so in underdeveloped parts of the world, the first thing we think of to supplement is iodine. Iodine supplements, outside of the iodized salt that is on most of our tables in the US, are readily available in health food stores. If for some reason you do suspect iodine insufficiency (for example, you have regularly consumed large quantities of foods that bind it and make it unavailable for use) and you are intent on supplementation, kelp is one of the best sources of natural organic iodine. It has been suggested that organic iodine is far better and more bioavailable than the inorganic iodine with which we supplement our table salt.

Another way to supplement iodine can be found in the form of a liquid that is applied to the bottom of the feet, by the name of Lugol's (aqueous) Iodine. The idea is that your skin will absorb the iodine it needs as you continue to apply it until the skin will no longer absorb it.

However, excess iodine can actually inhibit thyroid synthesis. The FDA's Recommended Daily Allowance of iodine is actually quite small, only 150 micrograms or 150 millionths of a gram, but it is estimated that the average American's daily intake is over 600 micrograms daily. Because we typically get plenty of iodine and its only function in the body is to synthesize thyroid hormone, it is recommended that iodine supplementation or consumption in food not exceed 600 mcg per day for extended periods. In addition, taking iodine supplements can be dangerous for patients with Graves disease (autoimmune hyperthyroidism) or 'hot' nodules of overactive thyroid. Before supplementing iodine, work with a medical provider to determine that your iodine levels are insufficient for normal thyroid function.

Tyrosine
Tyrosine is an amino acid that is also typically plentiful in our diets via animal protein or whole grains, fruits and legumes. All of these food sources are plentiful in the foods that support your

thyroid. If supplementation is needed, there are numerous supplements available in health food stores.

Vitamins

Vitamin A and vitamin E function together in the manufacture of thyroid hormone as well as in many other of your body's processes. The B vitamins B2 (riboflavin), B3 (niacin) and B6 (pyridoxine) are necessary for normal thyroid hormone manufacture, as is vitamin C. Lower levels of active thyroid hormone would be the result of a deficiency in any of these nutrients.

Minerals

There may be a correlation between hypothyroidism in the elderly and the fact that low zinc levels are also common in this population. Copper is another mineral essential for proper thyroid function. Calcium is indicated as hypothyroidism medication may cause bone loss. Consult your health care provider for recommended dosage.

All of the vitamins and minerals mentioned may be found in a single high-quality multi-vitamin and mineral preparation, although you may have to use a separate calcium supplement to get sufficient quantities.

Herbs

Herbal supplements that support thyroid function include milk thistle, which stimulates thyroid function and improves thyroid hormone conversion. Bladderwrack contains iodine, see a naturopath for a prescription after consultation to determine iodine levels. Coleus stimulates the release of thyroid hormone, also requires naturopathic prescription. Guggul contains guggulsterones, which exhibit thyroid-stimulating activity and requires a naturopathic prescription.

Other

The FDA requires thyroid extracts sold in health food stores to be free of thyroxine to prevent the serious consequences of overdose, for example, insomnia, severe anxiety, and heart disturbances. However, it is nearly impossible to remove all the hormone from the natural sources of thyroid extracts. Health-food-store thyroid preparations are basically milder preparations of natural thyroid. If you have mild hypothyroidism, these preparations may provide enough support to help you with your thyroid problem. If you begin to exhibit signs of hyperthyroidism, discontinue use of these preparations and seek medical consultation. In addition, most health-food store thyroid preparations include iodine, tyrosine and zinc as well. Please see the cautions associated with these substances before deciding to take these preparations outside the care of a doctor or naturopath.

Lifestyle changes

First and foremost, if you smoke, STOP! Do this for all the conventional reasons as well as to avoid compromising your thyroid function. While you are eliminating unhelpful habits, you might consider also limiting or eliminating caffeine and alcohol as well, as both have a negative effect on the metabolism.

Exercise

Exercise, particularly aerobic exercise, can be helpful in restoring normal thyroid function or avoiding thyroid disease in the first place. It is an irony that one of the symptoms of thyroid disease, both hypo- and hyperthyroidism, is fatigue. When you feel fatigued, it is nearly impossible to motivate yourself to exercise, of course. However, you will feel better overall if you can get past the reluctance and just do it. Even if it does not actually improve the thyroid condition (as no one has been able to determine how to make a non-functioning thyroid function again), it will still have other benefits that are worth pursuing.

Exercise both stimulates bodily function including that of thyroid hormone production and increases cell sensitivity to hormone activity. It is especially important in overweight hypothyroid individuals who are dieting, as the calorie restriction associated with dieting can suppress the metabolism in a circular feedback loop that will further exacerbate hypothyroidism, lowering the metabolism even further and so on. This effect is highly suspect in our current obesity epidemic and is the single most likely culprit in yo-yo dieting syndrome.

Light therapy

Light therapy in the form of getting 10 minutes of natural sunlight (without the filter of glasses or windows) per day stimulates the pineal gland, with beneficial effect to all the endocrine glands including the thyroid. Look toward but not directly at the sun, preferably early in the day, for the best benefit.

Self-care therapies

Self-care therapies that can be done at home with appropriate supervision of a professional therapist help to balance your energies and restore general health. They include biofeedback training and neurotherapy, various physical disciplines such as yoga, tai-chi and qigong and energy work on the throat chakra. You can also take a cool shower morning and evening to stimulate thyroid activity, or alternate hot and cold compresses to the throat, hot for 5 minutes followed by ice-cold for 30 seconds, for 3-5 repetitions. Hot/cold compress therapy should be repeated morning and evening for 5 days, and then morning only for 30 days.

Relaxation

Do not discount the value of relaxation. Our modern lives are so driven with work, frequently long commutes, child care and nurturing, and frenetic social obligations that we have lost the ability to simply relax. If you think that relaxing involves sipping a glass of wine or a cocktail while watching television, relaxation therapy is definitely for you. Long-term stress can cause suppression of the immune system, memory loss, decrease sexual drive, suppression of the immune system, rapid or irregular heartbeat, anxiety, irritability, depression, exaggeration of allergies, muscle tension, cancer, poor digestion, poor absorption of nutrients leading to nutritional deficiencies, skin disorders, back problems, increased cortisol levels and more. Does this sound familiar? Note the similarity between these symptoms and those of hypothyroidism.

There is a very simple method to determine whether an activity (or lack thereof) that you have chosen to relax is actually getting the job done: how does it make you feel? Whether you relax by taking a warm bath, perhaps with essential oils added or by taking a brisk walk, it should make you feel rested (or invigorated), give you an overall feeling of well-being and lift your mood. If it does not do that, it is not relaxation. Meditation is a great way to relax, but do not allow the perfect practice of the method to intimidate you. Simply go somewhere quiet, get physically comfortable, close your eyes and focus on your breathing. If you fall asleep, so much the better-you must need the rest!

Hydrotherapy

Contrast application to the neck and throat may stimulate thyroid function. Alternate three minutes hot with one minute cold, three times for one set. Daily therapy for two to three sets is recommended.

Other therapies

Acupuncture, detoxification (see below), cell therapy and magnetic field therapy may be helpful, either alone or in combination.

Symptom relief

Many of the symptoms of hypothyroidism can be relieved by treating the symptom itself, although these treatments may not address the underlying condition. For example, progesterone cream treatment can help symptoms associated with menstrual problems. The simple expedient of dressing in layers that you can remove or put on as necessary will alleviate sensitivity to cold or heat. Symptoms of fatigue, insomnia, depression, anxiety or stress can be relieved with nutrition, supplements, lifestyle and simple dietary adjustments (like avoiding stimulants and depressants such as caffeine and alcohol).

More meal ideas and recipes

A sample 7-day menu

Sunday

Breakfast - Mock California Eggs Benedict

Mid-morning snack - 1 piece of fruit

Lunch - Tuna salad served on a bed of quinoa or chickpeas, topped with crumbled feta cheese

Mid afternoon snack - Celery sticks with hummus or tahini

Dinner - Grilled lean meat or chicken. ½ C Quinoa with roasted pine nuts, stir-fried vegetables

Monday

Breakfast - Protein Shake, see Recipes below

Mid-morning snack - Handful of Trail Mix, see Recipes below

Lunch - Tomato Bisque see Recipes, below, 1 slice sourdough Rye toast with tahini,

Small mixed vegetable salad

Mid afternoon snack - Fruit salad: ½ apple, ¼ cup pineapple, 6 raspberries or blueberries, 2 tbsp natural organic yoghurt

Dinner - Poached fish with steamed mixed vegetables, seasoned with lemon and herbs.

Tuesday

Breakfast - ½ C steel-cut or old-fashioned oats, cooked to taste, ½ chopped apple. Oat, almond or rice milk. Add a small amount of pecans if desired

Mid-morning snack - 3-oz can of tuna packed in water or 2 hard-boiled eggs

Lunch - Greek salad (chopped cucumber, onion, green pepper, tomato and olive) with tuna or grilled chicken. See Recipes, below

Mid afternoon snack - Protein Shake

Dinner - Roast chicken with Roasted Root Vegetables, see Recipes below

Wednesday

Breakfast - Protein Shake

Mid-morning snack - Handful of nuts and seeds or Trail Mix

Lunch - Fiesta Chicken Soup, see Recipes, below. 1 serving baked blue corn tortilla chips

Mid afternoon snack - Green smoothie, see Recipes, below

Dinner - Grilled fish with Mediterranean Sauce, see Recipes, below, ½ C brown rice or quinoa

Thursday

Breakfast - ½ C high-protein muesli, blueberries or raspberries, Oat, almond or rice milk

Mid-morning snack - Protein Shake

Lunch - Open tuna salad sandwich on 1 slice sourdough rye. Small mixed-vegetable sandwich

Mid afternoon snack - 1 slice toast with grilled tomato, avocado and tuna or grilled chicken. Add beet greens if desired.

Dinner - Chicken Masala with curried vegetables, see Recipes, below, ½ C quinoa or brown rice

Friday

Breakfast - Protein shake, see Recipes below

Mid-morning snack - Piece of fruit, fruit juice or vegetable juice

Lunch - Large mixed vegetable salad topped with 3 oz of water-packed tuna or grilled chicken breast

Mid afternoon snack - Veggie burger or minced beef burger, dressed with lettuce, tomato, onion and mushrooms, on rye or mixed whole-grain bun

Dinner - Celery sticks and baby carrots with tahini or yogurt dip

Saturday

Breakfast - Oatmeal pancakes, see recipes below. Top with pureed banana or other tropical fruit and chopped pecans if desired. Green tea

Mid-morning snack - Small raw vegetable salad with 1 chopped hard-boiled egg and topped with crumbled feta

Lunch - Gazpacho, see Recipes, below. Served with small mixed-vegetable salad

Mid afternoon snack - Fruit salad

Dinner - Vegetarian chili, served with organic corn tortillas and homemade salsa, see Recipes, below

Recipes in the 7-day menu

Mock California eggs Benedict

1 piece sourdough rye bread, toasted and sliced in half

2 poached eggs

1 grilled tomato, halved before grilling

½ avocado, sliced

Arrange grilled tomato and sliced avocado evenly on toast halves. Top each with 1 poached egg. Savor slowly!

Nutritional Values

Servings: 2

Calories/Serving: 195

Total fat: 12.3 g

Sodium: 249.6 mg

Total Carbs 13.8 g

Dietary Fiber 4.4 g

Protein 8.8 g

Protein shake (three selections)

Protein shakes can contain from 250-600+ calories depending on what ingredients you use and how much of the preparation you consume. When using a shake for a snack rather than a meal, select those ingredients that keep it on the lower end of the scale, or cut the recipe in half, or share with a friend. You may calculate the calories of your favorite using any of several online services that have free recipe calorie calculators.

Shake #1: Thyroid support

1 oz goji juice

2-4 tsp protein powder (choose whatever kind you can tolerate other than soy)

2-3 tsp lecithin

1 T flaxseed or coconut oil

½ C berries (raspberries, blueberries, boysenberries or mixed) best choice

or

½ ripe banana, a few mango slices or other tropical fruit of your liking almond, oat or rice milk or water and/or ice to taste optional: 1 tsp chlorophyll or spirulina

Blend until frothy and all powders are thoroughly mixed in, thinning with milk or water until it is the consistency you like.

Shake #2 – Banana berry

2/3 cup unsweetened pear juice

1/2 banana, frozen

1/2 cup blackberries

1/2 cup of ice

1/2 cup of water

1 T extra dark cocoa powder

2 scoops of unflavored protein powder

Blend until protein powder is mixed thoroughly.

Shake #3 –Nutty fruit

For a creamier shake:

1 ½ cups almond milk

2 heaping tablespoons of brown rice protein powder

2 cups frozen mixed fruit

Blend and enjoy

Trail mix

Make your trail mix with the nuts and seeds that promote thyroid health, and avoid those that interfere with thyroid function. Add dried berries to taste, and if desired, add some dark chocolate chips or carob chips to make it a treat. Here's an example:

1 C pecans

1 C pumpkin seeds

½ C sunflower seeds

1 C dried cranberries

½ C golden raisins

1 oz unsweetened coconut flakes

Mix thoroughly and enjoy in ¼ C servings. Although they contain nutrients that are very good for you (even essential), nuts, seeds and dried berries are high in calories, so enjoy in moderation! Choose raw, unsalted nuts and seeds, and organic ingredients where possible. Nutrition analysis does not include optional chocolate or carob chips.

Nutritional Values

Servings: 22

Calories/Serving: 108

Total fat: 6.1g

Sodium: 21.3 mg

Total Carbs 13.2 g

Dietary Fiber 1.9 g

Protein 1.7 g

Tomato bisque

2 tablespoons extra-virgin olive oil

1 onion, chopped

3 cloves garlic, minced

1 (28-ounce) can whole tomatoes, with liquid

1/4-1/2 cup roasted garlic tomato paste

2 cups vegetable or organic chicken stock

2-2 1/2 cups butternut squash, peeled and diced

Salt and ground pepper to taste

2 tablespoons fresh basil, chopped

1/2 teaspoon dried thyme

1 to 1 1/4 cups nonfat yogurt

Several dashes of Tabasco or other hot pepper sauce

In a large saucepan, sauté onions and garlic in oil over medium-low heat until soft and golden. Add tomatoes, tomato paste, chicken stock, butternut squash, salt, pepper, basil and thyme. Bring to a boil, then reduce heat. Partially cover and simmer for about 30-35 minutes, or until squash is fork-tender. Puree the soup in a blender, then pour back into the saucepan. Stir in nonfat yogurt, splash in the hot pepper sauce, and taste for seasoning. Heat the soup just to a boil, then ladle into bowls. Garnish with sliced basil leaves or minced parsley.

Nutritional Values

Servings: 6

Calories/Serving: 167

Total fat: 5.1 g

Sodium: 955.4 mg

Total Carbs 29.5 g

Dietary Fiber 1.4 g

Protein 4.8 g

Roasted root vegetables

1 T olive oil

1 red onion, sliced

4 cloves garlic, peeled and cut in half

2 carrots, peeled and diced

1 beet, peeled and diced

1 yam or sweet potato, peeled and diced

2 parsnips, peeled and diced

1 t dried rosemary

1 t dried thyme

1 pinch salt

1/2 t black pepper

1 T balsamic vinegar, optional

Preheat oven to 375°F. Spray a baking pan or cookie sheet with nonstick cooking spray. Combine all ingredients in a mixing bowl; toss to combine. Place mixture in pan. Bake 30 minutes, turning vegetables every 10 minutes until vegetables are tender and slightly browned. Drizzle with balsamic vinegar before serving.

Nutritional Values

Servings: 8

Calories/Serving: 82

Total fat: 1.9 g

Sodium: 36.6mg

Total Carbs 15.8 g

Dietary Fiber 3.2 g

Protein 1.4 g

Fiesta chicken soup

1 tsp olive oil

Cooked chicken, in bite size pieces (about 10oz) You can use leftover roast or grilled chicken, or canned chicken breast

1 can fat free refried beans (16oz)

1 can diced tomatoes with green chilies (14.5 oz) or substitute your favorite salsa

1 can yellow sweet corn (12 oz) or equal amount fresh or frozen

1 cup brown rice, cooked

1-2 cloves fresh garlic, minced

1 tsp adobo seasoning (found in the Latin foods section of your grocer)

1-2 C water, enough to dilute soup to taste

Add salt and pepper to taste (to lower the sodium content of this soup, substitute fresh ingredients for canned and do not add extra salt)

Nutritional Values

Servings: 6

Calories/Serving: 213

Total fat: 2.3 g

Sodium: 614.3 mg

Total Carbs 28.9 g

Dietary Fiber 6 g

Protein 18.1 g

Green smoothie

Green smoothies can be made with your own favorite fruits and vegetables, taking care to choose those that support thyroid function from the list in the previous section of this book. Lower the sugar content by choosing vegetables rather than fruit; add cilantro and parsley for detoxification; and experiment! As calorie content will vary according to what you choose, we will not attempt to provide it here. An essential ingredient is Swiss chard, which supports thyroid function and will indeed make your smoothie green! Don't worry, it does not taste 'green.' Adding sufficient fruit such as banana, mango or pineapple to sweeten it up a bit will make almost any combination palatable. Add protein powder of your choice to increase nutritional value, and if you prefer a thicker drink, add some crushed ice. Blend and enjoy. If you happen to create a combination that you don't like, keep adding ingredients until it is more to your taste. Be fearless!

Grilled fish with Mediterranean sauce

You may use any type of fish you prefer with this sauce, and it is just as good baked as grilled. If you happen to not particularly care for fish but know you should be eating more for heart health, this sauce is a delicious way to make it tasty enough for the most finicky eater.

2 teaspoon olive oil

1 large onion, sliced

1 can (16 oz.) whole tomatoes, drained (reserve juice) and coarsely chopped

1 bay leaf

1 clove garlic, minced

1/2 cup reserved tomato juice, from canned tomatoes

1/4 cup lemon juice

1/2 cup orange juice

1 tablespoon fresh grated orange peel

1 teaspoon fennel seeds, crushed

1/2 teaspoon dried oregano, crushed

1/2 teaspoon dried thyme, crushed

1/2 teaspoon dried basil, crushed

Black pepper to taste

1 lb. fish fillets

Heat oil in large non-stick skillet. Add onion and sauté over moderate heat 5 minutes or until soft. Add all remaining ingredients except fish. Stir well and simmer 30 minutes, uncovered.

When about 10 minutes remains, grill fish or

Arrange fish in 10x6" baking dish; cover with sauce. Bake uncovered at 375º F about 15 minutes or until fish flakes easily.

Yield: 4 servings--Serving Size: 4 oz fillet with sauce

Nutritional Values

Servings: 4

Calories/Serving: 225.5

Total fat: 4.4 g

Sodium: 277 mg

Total Carbs 17.3 g

Dietary Fiber 2.5 g

Protein 29.4 g

Chicken Masala

1/4 t black pepper

2 T whole wheat pastry flour (or substitute gluten-free thickener of your choice)

1/2 c fat free chicken broth

Juice of 1/4 lemon wedge

1 c fresh sliced mushrooms

2 (5 oz) chicken breasts, boneless, skinless

1/2 c Masala wine

Nonstick spray

Mix pepper and flour together. Dredge chicken breasts in flour mixture.

Heat a heavy skillet over medium heat. Spray with non-stick spray and brown both sides of chicken. Remove browned chicken and reserve.

To skillet, add wine, lemon juice, broth and mushrooms. Stir to toss and heat through. Add browned chicken. Cover and simmer for 10-15 minutes until chicken is cooked through, turning occasionally. Uncover and simmer for 2-3 minutes more, or until sauce reduces and thickens.

2 servings

Nutritional Values

Servings: 2

Calories/Serving: 217

Total fat: 2.1 g

Sodium:217.9 mg

Total Carbs 8.7 g

Dietary Fiber 1.6 g

Protein 35.2 g

Oatmeal pancakes

1/2 cup dry oatmeal

1/2 cup fat free cottage cheese

4 egg whites

1/2 tsp baking powder

1/2 tsp vanilla

Blend egg whites first until you have a foamy liquid. Add everything except the oats. Once you have a smooth liquid, add the oats and blend for only a little bit, you want the batter to be a little bumpy. Let the batter sit for a couple minutes, to thicken up a bit. If desired, you may add blueberries or other fruit to the batter at this point.

Cook in a pan or griddle coated with no stick cooking spray. Makes about six 4-5" pancakes.

You may top with fruit, jam or syrup if you wish and can afford the calories. The original of this recipe called for a packet or two of Stevia or artificial sweetener; however the author has never missed the sweeter flavor, and has usually topped the pancakes with fruit compote.

Nutritional Values

Servings: 6 (1 pancake each)

Calories/Serving: 47.5

Total fat: .5 g

Sodium: 146.1 mg

Total Carbs 4.6 g

Dietary Fiber 0.7 g

Protein 5.6 g

Gazpacho (chilled vegetable soup)

Here's a Spanish-influence vegetable soup that is appropriate for omnivores and vegans alike.

1 slice bakery bread (about 1 cup) without crust; torn into bite-sized pieces

1/2 red onion

1 yellow or red bell pepper

2 cloves garlic

1 banana pepper

1 cucumber

5 large tomatoes (about 1 1/2 pounds)

1-2 tablespoons red wine vinegar

1/2 teaspoon black pepper

Place the bread into a mixing bowl, cover with one cup of cold water and soak for five minutes.

Roughly chop onion; remove seeds from peppers and roughly chop; peel cucumber and cut into fourths. Place the onion, peppers, and garlic into the bowl of a food processor, pulse three or four times. Add the cucumbers and tomatoes to food processor and pulse a few more times.

Squeeze excess liquid from the bread and add the wet bread to the soup mixture. Process for 20 seconds. Add vinegar and pepper to taste.

Garnish with chopped herbs, diced avocado, or grilled corn.

Makes 6 one cup servings.

Nutritional Values

Servings: 6 (1 cup each)

Calories/Serving: 89

Total fat: .6 g

Sodium: 96.3 mg

Total Carbs 18.4 g

Dietary Fiber2.4 g

Protein 2.2 g

Vegetarian chili

1 can black beans

2 cans butter beans (large)

1 or 2 cans stewed or Mexican-style tomatoes (by taste preference)

1 can fat-free chili beans or pintos

2 cups mushrooms, whole or halved

1.5 cups yams or sweet potatoes, cubed

1 onion (white) diced.

1 cup or more of sliced okra

1 red onion for garnish if desired

6 servings

You can reduce the sodium in this recipe by cooking your own dried beans without salt and adding 1½ C of each variety per can in the recipe; by choosing no-salt-added canned tomatoes, or both.

Nutritional Values

Servings: 6

Calories/Serving: 194

Total fat: 1.2 g

Sodium: 660 mg

Total Carbs 41.2 g

Dietary Fiber 10.3 g

Protein 9.1 g

Homemade salsa

3 large fresh tomatoes*

1 medium onion

1/4 bunch of cilantro (use more or less depending on your taste)

Juice of half a lemon

1/2 teaspoon of minced garlic

1 tsp of salt

2 jalapenos (or more if you prefer it hotter)

Optional ingredients (not included in nutritional analysis)

Half a cucumber, peeled and diced

1 avocado, peeled and diced

Wash tomatoes and cilantro. Dice tomatoes, onions; chop cilantro, jalapenos, and the optional ingredients (avocado, cucumber). Combine all ingredients in a bowl with salt, garlic and lemon juice.**

* To roast your tomatoes for great flavor:

Pre-heat skillet on medium high heat. Place whole tomatoes in the pan and toast, turning it until the skin begins to break and split apart. Remove from heat and continue as above.

**If you prefer smooth salsa as opposed to chunky, pulse in food processor until it is the consistency desired.

Nutritional Values

Servings: 8

Calories/Serving: 22.5

Total fat: .3 g

Sodium: 297.7 mg

Total Carbs 5.9 g

Dietary Fiber 1.6 g

Protein 0.9 g

As you can see, it is rather easy to find tasty and healthful recipes that support thyroid function as well as paying attention to the requirements of other health issues, such as lower calories, lower sodium, dairy-free and gluten-free.   Vegetarians and vegans should take care to rely less on tofu and other soy products, instead substituting other legumes for the animal proteins in these recipes. Adding legumes to the grains suggested completes the protein (i.e., combines to provide all essential amino acids) and provides plenty of it for those who prefer not to consume animal proteins.

Hypothyroidism and exercise

Always consult a healthcare professional before beginning an exercise program, particularly if you have been sedentary for quite some time.

If you are suffering from hypothyroidism and especially if your symptoms include fatigue, sluggishness, aching muscles and joints and lack of motivation to exercise, this may be the most challenging part of a natural therapy for you. It is easy enough to say you will feel better if you exercise, and indeed you will. However, you must first summon the mental energy to overcome your symptoms and do it.

One of the best exercises to start with if you have these symptoms or have been sedentary for some time and are perhaps seriously overweight, is walking. Even heart patients, who are cautioned not to raise their heart rate too high or are on medication to prevent it, can walk, if only a few steps at first. We will leave it to your doctor to tell you how much and how often, but following are some goals and suggested exercises that will be beneficial to your entire body, not just your thyroid. The author can attest that you can lose weight and get more fit without medication, having shed 45 pounds just by changing eating habits, paying more attention to serving size, and beginning an exercise program. You can do it, too!

Begin simply by walking as many steps as you can, every day. At first, this may mean just walking down the driveway to your mailbox. If you are consistent, you will find that you are able as the days and weeks go by to walk further and faster. Keep it up, you may become addicted to it! By the way, you don't have to walk fast to get some benefit. Walking fast or walking long, both will burn calories and help shed weight, which in turn will give you more energy and more motivation.

It is now known that adults should get at least 30 minutes of exercise a day, preferably that raises the heart rate to a level that lets you know you have exerted yourself, but not to leave you gasping for air. It is also now known that you do not have to do this all at once. If you can find even 10 minutes a few times a day to walk, climb stairs, dance or otherwise move vigorously, you will reap the benefits of better health. Choose activities that you enjoy; that way it will be a pleasure, not a chore. Make your household chores count, too. If you need to mop the floor, do it with vigor! Heavy housework is considered aerobic activity. Walk your dog, dance with your child, whatever it takes to move, 10 minutes at a time, 3 times a day.

Strength training, that is, lifting a moderate amount of weight or using your body as in squats, pushups or planks, is also important for total health. If you do not use your muscles, they grow progressively weaker, but remember to start slowly if you must. Doing curls with a standard can of vegetables is better than doing nothing at all.

A word about warming up and stretching. You may have seen runners stretching before they start running, calling it a warm-up. This is as likely to cause injury as not, as cold muscles tear rather than stretch. It is most beneficial to warm up by doing a slower version of the aerobic exercise you are about to enjoy or a different but still moderate aerobic activity. For example, if you are going to go on a vigorous walk, start a little slower to warm up. Or perhaps you could jog slowly in place for a few minutes before running. After a few minutes, if you feel the need to stretch your muscles before continuing, you may safely do so as they are now warm. It is always a good idea to cool down with some stretches to avoid muscle aches after vigorous exercise.

You may need to start out by establishing the habit of exercise. It is commonly believed that it takes 21 days to establish a habit. After that time, do not be surprised if you find yourself wanting more or more varied exercise, and that is a good thing! Before you know it, you'll be swimming, cycling, hiking or playing tennis—who knows, you might even decide to climb a mountain! It's all good.

Benefits of regular exercise:

- Boosts immune function
- Lowers blood pressure
- Improves circulation
- Increases bone mass and strengthens bones
- Lowers 'bad' cholesterol
- Boosts 'good' cholesterol
- Reduces stress
- Lifts depression
- Makes your dog and your kids happy!
- It's fun!

Ways to add movement to your daily life:

- Park your car further from the entrance
- Better yet, leave the car at home and walk to work or for errands
- Take the stairs most of the time
- Buy a pedometer for motivation
- Take a brisk walk on your lunch hour—invite your co-workers and make it a party
- Play chase with your children

- Buy a hula hoop or jump rope and indulge your inner child
- Dance while cooking dinner or doing laundry
- In inclement weather, go mall-walking
- Buy a small medicine ball and play with it while you watch TV. (You can get one as light as 5 lbs.)
- Take a bike ride or go swimming with your family

The more playful you can make your exercise and added movement, the more it will lighten your mood and the more you will want to do it.

Resources

Information about the thyroid and illnesses of the thyroid; health tips, weight loss and alternative therapies:

American Thyroid Association: www.thyroid.org/index.html

Medical Encyclopedia:
www.nlm.nih.gov/medlineplus/ency/article/000353.htm
(Hypothyroidism)

http://www.nlm.nih.gov/medlineplus/ency/article/000371.htm
(Hashimoto's Disease)

WebMD: www.webmd.com/a-to-z-guides/hypothyroidism-topic-overview

Thyroid-Info.com: www.thyroid-info.com/index.htm

STOP The Thyroid Madness:
http://www.stopthethyroidmadness.com/

Dr Rind.com: http://www.drrind.com/therapies/metabolic-therapy

Dr Broda Barnes: http://www.brodabarnes.org /

Weight loss: www.livinghealthweightloss.com

Healthnotes:

http://www.vitamins.com/vf/healthnotes/HN75_english/Index/All_Index.htm

WholeHealthMD.com:

http://www.wholehealthmd.com/ME2/dirmod.asp?sid=17E09E7CFFF640448FFB0B4FC1B7FEF0&type=AWHN&nm=Reference+Library&mod=Home&style=1

Herbal Medicine Website: http://www.herbs2000.com/

Vitamin & Mineral Website:
http://lpi.oregonstate.edu/infocenter/

Nutrition Website: http://www.nutritiondata.com /

More recipes and tips for nutritional support:

The Hypothyroidism Solution Cookbook by Duncan Cappicianno, N.D.

Appendix A – Quotes

Thyroid function tests and their applicability to the individual:

Anthony Toft and Geoffrey Beckett BMJ 2003 (8 February); 326:295-296

"It is extraordinary that more than 100 years since the first description of the treatment of hypothyroidism and the current availability of refined diagnostic tests, debate is continuing about its diagnosis and management."

C Meier, P Trittibach et al, "Serum thyroid stimulating hormone in assessment of severity of tissue hypothyroidism in patients with overt primary thyroid failure: cross sectional survey" British Medical Journal, 2003 (8 February); 326:311-312

"TSH is a poor measure for estimating the clinical and metabolic severity of primary overt thyroid failure. This is in sharp contrast to the high diagnostic accuracy of TSH measurement for early diagnosis of hypothyroidism.

Joseph H Keffer, "Preanalytical Considerations in Testing Thyroid Function"

Clinical Chemistry 1996; 42(1):125-134

"The application of population-based norms is inappropriately wide when applied to individuals. Each person has a narrow range of fluctuation of T4, even with seasonal or annual study."

Reference Ranges for thyroid function tests are based on statistical averages. They are not based on standards of biological activity at different levels of thyroid hormones. This is not a problem in itself provided that the circumstances of the individual are always considered. The particular issue for thyroid patients is that an individual's thyroid hormone levels do not naturally move over the whole Reference Range. Individual thyroid hormone levels are confined to narrow personalized ranges around the so called Set Point. Being in this personal range is important.

Stig Andersen et al, "Narrow Individual Variations in Serum T4 and T3 in Normal Subjects: A Clue to the Understanding of Subclinical Thyroid Disease"

Journal of Clinical Endocrinology and Metabolism, 2002 March; 87(3):1068-72

"High individuality causes laboratory reference ranges to be insensitive to changes in test results that are significant for the individual."

LM Demers PhD FACB, CA Spencer PhD FACB, "NACB: Laboratory Support for the Diagnosis and Monitoring of Thyroid Disease"

The National Academy of Clinical Biochemistry Laboratory Medicine Practice Guidelines, 2002

http://www.nacb.org/lmpg/thyroid_lmpg_pub.stm

"It is now well documented that hypothyroid patients have serum FT4 values in the upper third of the reference interval when the L-T4 replacement dose is titered [adjusted] to bring the serum TSH into the therapeutic target range (0.5-2.0 mIU/L)."

"...Also, as shown in Figure 2, serum TSH values are diagnostically misleading during transition periods of unstable thyroid status, such as occurs in the early phase of treating hyper- or hypothyroidism or changing the dose of L-T4. Specifically, it takes 6-12 weeks for pituitary TSH secretion to re-equilibrate to the new thyroid hormone status. These periods of unstable thyroid status may also occur following an episode of thyroiditis, including post-partum thyroiditis when discordant TSH and FT4 values may also be encountered."

Dr Lawrence C Wood, "TSH: A new "normal"?: New guidelines from the National Academy of Clinical Biochemistry (NACB)".

Thyroid Federation International, Thyrobulletin, Spring 2002; 5(1): 9

"Dr. Carole Spencer from USC Medical Center recently reviewed new research indicating that the normal range for TSH is actually much lower than the range presently accepted in virtually all medical laboratories."

American Association of Clinical Endocrinologists, "New Campaign Urges People to "Think Thyroid" at Critical Life Stages and Get Tested", Thyroid Awareness Month 2001, Jan 2001

"AACE encourages patients whose TSH is outside the normal range (.5-5.0 µU/ml) to see an endocrinologist for treatment and thyroid disease management. Even though a TSH level between 3.0 and 5.0 µU/ml is in the normal range, it should be considered suspect since it may signal a case of evolving thyroid underactivity."

Drs Colin M Dayan, Ponnusamy Saravanan, & Graham Bayly, "Whose normal thyroid function is better – yours or mine?"

The Lancet, 3 Aug 2002; 360(9330): 353

"A typical (statistical) reference range for thyroid-stimulating hormone (TSH) in many laboratories is around 0.2-5.5 mU/L. [NB: This reference range has been significantly lowered in the years since this publication.] However, the 20-year longitudinal Whickham survey indicated that individuals with TSH values greater than 2.0 mU/L have an increased risk of developing overt hypothyroidism over the next 20 years."

More Books by John McArthur

Hypothyroidism
Hypothyroidism: The Hypothyroidism Solution. Hypothyroidism Natural Treatment and Hypothyroidism Diet for Under Active Or Slow Thyroid, Causing Weight Loss Problems, Fatigue, Cardiovascular Disease. John McArthur (Author), Cheri Merz (Editor)

Fibromyalgia And Chronic Fatigue
Fibromyalgia And Chronic Fatigue: A Step-By-Step Guide For Fibromyalgia Treatment And Chronic Fatigue Syndrome Treatment. Includes Fibromyalgia Diet And Chronic Fatigue Diet And Lifestyle Guidelines. John McArthur (Author), Cheri Merz (Editor)

Yeast Infection
Candida Albicans: Yeast Infection Treatment. Treat Yeast Infections With This Home Remedy. The Yeast Infection Cure. John McArthur (Author)

Heart Disease
Hypertension - High Blood Pressure: How To Lower Blood Pressure Permanently In 8 Weeks Or Less, The Hypertension Treatment, Diet and Solution. John McArthur (Author)

Cholesterol Myth: Lower Cholesterol Won't Stop Heart Disease.

Healthy Cholesterol Will. Cholesterol Recipe Book & Cholesterol Diet. Lower Cholesterol Naturally Keep Cholesterol Healthy. John McArthur (Author), Cheri Merz (Editor)

Heart Disease Prevention and Reversal: How To Prevent, Cure and Reverse Heart Disease Naturally For A Healthy Heart. John McArthur (Author)

Diabetes

Diabetes Diet: Diabetes Management Options. Includes a Diabetes Diet Plan with Diabetic Meals and Natural Diabetes Food, Herbs and Supplements for Total Diabetes Control. Delicious Recipes. John McArthur (Author), Corinne Watson (Editor)

Diabetes Cooking: 93 Diabetes Recipes for Breakfast, Lunch, Dinner, Snacks and Smoothies. A Guide to Diabetes Foods to Help You Prepare Healthy Delicious ... Diabetic Meals and Natural Diabetes Food) John McArthur (Author), Corinne Watson (Editor)

Stress and Anxiety

From Stressful to Successful in 4 Easy Steps: Stress at Work? Stress in Relationship? Be Stress Free. End Stress and Anxiety. Excellent Stress Management, Stress Control and Stress Relief Techniques. John McArthur (Author)

Anxiety and Panic Attacks: Anxiety Management. Anxiety Relief.

The Natural And Drug Free Relief For Anxiety Attacks, Panic Attacks And Panic Disorder. John McArthur (Author), Cheri Merz (Editor)

Back and Neck Pain
The 15 Minute Back Pain and Neck Pain Management Program: Back Pain and Neck Pain Treatment and Relief 15 Minutes a Day No Surgery No Drugs. Effective, Quick and Lasting Back and Neck Pain Relief. John McArthur (Author)

Arthritis
Arthritis: Arthritis Relief for Osteoarthritis, Rheumatoid Arthritis, Gout, Psoriatic Arthritis, and Juvenile Arthritis. Follow The Arthritis Diet, Cure and Treatment Free Yourself From The Pain. John McArthur (Author)

Depression
How to Break the Grip of Depression: Read How Robert Declared War On Depression ... And Beat It! John McArthur (Author)

Pregnancy
Pregnancy Nutrition: Pregnancy Food. Pregnancy Recipes. Healthy Pregnancy Diet. Pregnancy Health. Pregnancy Eating and Recipes. Nutritional Tips and 63 Delicious Recipes for Moms-to-Be. Corinne Watson (Author), John McArthur (Author)

Pregnancy and Childbirth: Expecting a Baby. Pregnancy Guide. Pregnancy What to Expect. Pregnancy Health. Pregnancy Eating and Recipes. Cheri Merz (Author), John McArthur (Author)

Allergies

Allergy Free: Fast Effective Drug-free Relief for Allergies. Allergy Diet. Allergy Treatments. Allergy Remedies. Natural Allergy Relief. John McArthur (Author), Cheri Merz (Editor)

Printed in Great Britain
by Amazon.co.uk, Ltd.,
Marston Gate.